JONAS SALK

Discoverer of the Polio Vaccine

— P E O P L E   T O   K N O W —

JONAS SALK

Discoverer of the Polio Vaccine

Carmen Bredeson

ENSLOW PUBLISHERS,INC.

Bloy St. and Ramsey Ave.   P.O. Box 38
Box 777   Aldershot
Hillside, N.J. 07205   Hants GU12 6BP
U.S.A.   U.K.

Library of Congress Cataloging-in-Publication Data

Bredeson, Carmen.
    Jonas Salk : discoverer of the polio vaccine / Carmen Bredeson.
       p. cm.— (People to know)
    Includes bibliographical references and index.
    Summary: Discusses the life and accomplishments of Jonas Salk,
including his discovery of the vaccine against polio and his work on
influenza and AIDS.
    ISBN 0-89490-415-9
    1. Salk, Jonas, 1914- —Juvenile literature. 2. Virologists-
-United States—Biography—Juvenile literature. 3. Poliomyelitis
vaccine—Juvenile literature. [1. Salk, Jonas, 1914-
2. Scientists. 3. Poliomyelitis vaccine.] I. Title. II. Series.
QR31.S25B74 1993
610'.92—dc20
[B]
                                      93-12097
                                       CIP
                                       AC

Printed in the United States of America

10 9 8 7 6 5 4 3 2 1

Illustration Credits:
James A. Cox, p. 6; Library of Congress, p. 15; March of Dimes Birth
Defects Foundation, pp. 9, 33, 34, 38, 41, 44, 51, 55, 63, 71, 73, 77, 78,
80, 85, 93; National Archives, pp. 30, 57; San Diego Union/Jerry Rife, p.
90.

Cover Illustration:
James A. Cox

Contents

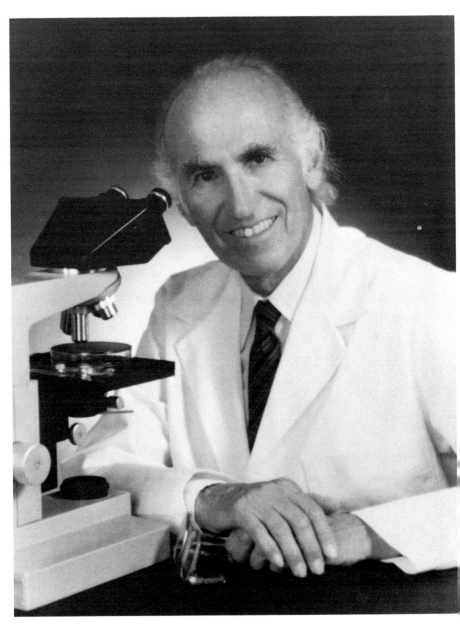

Jonas Salk, M.D.

1

April 12, 1955

Doctor Jonas Salk made his way slowly onto the stage at the University of Michigan's Rackham Hall. He sat down and straightened the papers in his lap. As the cameras and microphones were being adjusted, the forty-year-old research scientist peered into the audience to see if he could get a glimpse of his wife and three young sons. He had spent so little time with them recently. Thankfully Peter, Darrell, and Jonathan Salk had not been infected with the polio virus. During the previous summer of 1954, more than 38,000 others had not been as fortunate.

For the past four years Salk and his associates at the University of Pittsburgh had worked day and night to find a vaccine to combat polio. Every year more and more cases of the crippling and sometimes fatal disease were reported. And most often the victims of the disease were young children. Since polio was transmitted from person to person, swimming pools, movie theaters, and even schools had been closed in an attempt to halt the spread of the virus.

In spite of the precautions, ambulances lined up in communities all across America to deliver the latest polio cases to local hospitals. Once inside the polio wards, patients of all ages suffered as the virus attacked their bodies. Affected arms and legs were often bent into unnatural positions and held there by rigid cramped muscles. Many of the beds were occupied by children who were too young to understand what was happening. They could only cry in pain and fear for their mothers and fathers. This terrible suffering had to be stopped.

Just one year ago, after endless experiments in his laboratory, Salk had finally been ready to administer an experimental vaccine to a large number of volunteers. Nearly two million school children in towns all across America agreed to be "Polio Pioneers" and help test the vaccine. That massive field trial had taken place in the spring of 1954. And today, April 12, 1955, the results would be made public.

Jonas Salk was as uninformed as the 500 people in the audience, for he didn't know the outcome of the field trials either. He had not been part of the team that evaluated the confidential data as it arrived from 127 vaccination centers. Did his vaccine protect against

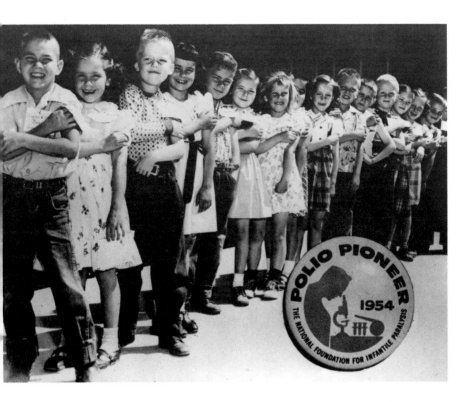

These children were among the many "Polio Pioneers" who helped test Dr. Salk's vaccine in 1954.

polio? Had there been bad reactions or even fatalities as a result of the vaccine? The last year had been a long one for Salk as he waited for the answers to these questions.

The lights in the auditorium dimmed, and Doctor Thomas Francis, Jr., director of the Poliomyelitis Vaccine Evaluation Center, stepped up to the microphone. A hush fell over the crowd as he began to speak. Francis opened his report with the words "the vaccine works!"[1] By the end of the hour-and-a-half report it was evident that the vaccine was not only effective but was also safe. In the auditorium applause erupted and the audience came to its feet. A smile spread across Salk's face as he rose from his seat to acknowledge the ovation.

Reporters raced from the room to file their stories, and radio and television announcers prepared bulletins to inform the public of the wonderful news. Doctor Jonas Salk became an instant hero. Radio and television broadcasts proclaimed the success of the vaccine. Church bells rang, horns honked, and people cheered in response to the thrilling news. A terrible disease could now be stopped.

Children would once again be free to swim, play, and go to the movies. Parents felt a profound sense of relief, for their lives would no longer be governed by fear. In the days that followed, thousands of letters and telegrams were sent to Dr. Salk. His phone rang from early morning until late at night with people calling to offer their congratulations and thanks.

Instead of printing a daily total of new polio cases, the newspapers turned their attention to Jonas Salk. The quiet scholarly scientist was suddenly assaulted on all sides by requests for interviews. Radio and television producers asked him to appear on their programs. Hollywood even wanted to make a movie about his life.

Many were interested in knowing more about the man behind the vaccine. Where did he grow up? What led him to go into the field of research? Doctor Jonas Salk really just wanted to spend some time with his family and get back to work in the laboratory. But first he would have to answer the questions that the American public was asking.

2

Salk's Early Years

On October 28, 1914, Russian immigrants Daniel and Dolly Salk welcomed their first child, Jonas, into the world. Like so many others, the Salks had moved to America in search of a better way of life. Daniel Salk worked hard at his job in the clothing industry. Even though they lived in a run-down New York City tenement, the Salks had high expectations for their family.

When Jonas was two years old a terrible epidemic of polio swept across the United States. There were at least 27,000 cases of the disease reported, and over 9,000 of the victims lived in New York City. Public hysteria increased as new polio cases continued to be diagnosed during that long summer in 1916.

Since children were polio's most frequent victims,

they were also looked upon as carriers of the disease. Sick children were taken to area hospitals, separated from their parents, and put into isolation. Sometimes their toys and blankets were burned in an attempt to keep the polio germs from spreading. Homes where the disease struck were often quarantined, and people were not allowed to enter or leave the premises.

During those early epidemics the experts could not explain how polio was transmitted. Everything was suspected of spreading the sickness, including dogs and cats, fleas, ticks, water, and even air itself. Houses were cleaned with strong soap, and trash was removed from the streets every day. Doors and windows were kept tightly closed, and frightened families stayed inside to try to escape the disease.[1]

Gradually, as the fall season with its cooler weather approached, the number of new polio cases decreased. People hoped that the epidemic was finally over. Even in warmer southern states, polio was almost always a summer illness. As the weather got cooler, polio seemed to disappear entirely. Life returned to normal, and the disease was all but forgotten during the long winter months.

Then, with the arrival of summer and the return of warm temperatures, polio once again struck. Case after case was reported during the hot months of 1917. This pattern of summer epidemics would continue for nearly forty years as the medical community studied the baffling illness.

During the frightening epidemics no one in the Salk household, which now included Jonas' brothers Lee and Herman, became infected with polio. As the family's financial situation began to improve, the Salks were able to move to a better apartment building in the Bronx, another New York City neighborhood. There they lived among other Jewish families whose older members often spoke with the foreign accents of their distant homelands.

Jonas was a thin dark-haired boy who went to elementary school near his home and made very good grades in all of his subjects. When he was just twelve years old he was given the opportunity to attend Townsend Harris High School for gifted boys. Students were enrolled there only if they agreed to work very hard and finish high school in three years instead of four.

Jonas had no trouble with the difficult courses offered at the special public school. He loved to read and listen to music, and he decided that he wanted to become a lawyer. Once when someone asked him about his future, Jonas said that "someday I shall grow up and do something in my own way, without anyone telling me how."[2]

By the time he was fifteen years old, Jonas graduated from Townsend Harris. His next step was to register at City College of New York to take the pre-law classes that

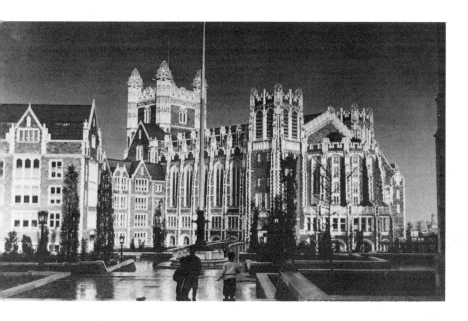

Jonas Salk registered at City College of New York when he was only fifteen years old. At first, Salk planned to study law.

would prepare him for law school. During his four years at City College, Jonas took a few science courses that interested him very much. Except for one class in physics in high school, Jonas had not studied science before.

Suddenly Salk discovered a new world as he explored the complex nature of living things. His brief introduction to science left him longing to know more about this mysterious and wonderful field. As his college graduation approached in 1934, Jonas decided that law school no longer interested him. He planned, instead, to enter medical school and become a doctor.

3

Medical School

The Great Depression was in full swing as Jonas Salk enrolled at the New York University School of Medicine in 1934. Thousands of people had lost their jobs, and extra money was scarce. Many families didn't have enough cash to buy groceries, let alone to send their children to college.

Mr. and Mrs. Salk borrowed money to help pay for their son's first year of medical school. During the following year, because he made excellent grades, Jonas was given several scholarships to help him financially. He also worked part-time to make extra spending money.

During his second year in medical school, Jonas did not take any regular classes, but instead, worked full-time in a laboratory. While employed there he learned about the science of biochemistry, which is the study of the chemical processes in the lives of plants and animals. He was good at making the detailed observations that were necessary to work in research. As Salk's medical education continued, he began to turn toward the analytical world of the laboratory and away from the traditional clinical role of doctors.

His fellow medical students criticized Salk for his choice because a great deal of money could be made as a private physician. Researchers, on the other hand, were usually underpaid and their work involved long hours of tedious experimentation. Certainly research was not a very glamorous profession. Most medical students were anxious to graduate and become successful practitioners of medicine.

During Salk's senior year, each student was allowed to spend two months doing elective work in a chosen field. Jonas naturally asked for a laboratory assignment and selected Dr. Thomas Francis, Jr., as his mentor or special teacher. Francis was one of the best known microbiologists in the United States and had discovered one of the viruses that causes influenza.

Historically, influenza has been a very serious illness. In the 1918–1919 pandemic, which is a worldwide epidemic, more than twenty-two million people died from problems associated with influenza. The disease spread into all walks of life so that no one was safe.

The situation became so desperate that New York state passed a law making it illegal to sneeze or cough in public if one's face was not covered with a handkerchief. Face masks became popular, and large public gatherings were discouraged.

Anxious people were willing to try any home remedy in an attempt to ward off the disease. Some people wore garlic or bags of camphor around their necks. The strong fumes were thought to drive away influenza germs. Others wore vinegar packs on their stomachs, tied cucumber slices to their ankles, or ate red pepper sandwiches. In spite of the useless precautions that some took, the spread of influenza could not be stopped.[1]

The influenza pandemic, which struck at the end of World War I, also took a huge toll among the soldiers who were involved in the fighting. As thousands of men died overseas, influenza claimed the lives of more than 500,000 Americans on the homefront. These were the years before the discovery of antibiotics.[2] Even though antibiotics such as penicillin and sulfa have no effect on the viral disease of influenza, they can be used to treat secondary bacterial infections such as pneumonia that killed so many flu victims in the past.

In spite of modern medicine, however, influenza is still a serious threat today. In 1987 alone, 33,464 Americans died from complications of influenza. The numbers rose to 37,674 in 1989, and even higher in 1990—when 39,857 deaths were reported.[3]

Dr. Thomas Francis had more experience in the field of virology than most of his peers. Salk's mentor was one of the few scientists who believed that an inactivated or killed virus vaccine could be developed that would protect people against illnesses such as influenza and polio. This possibility interested Jonas Salk because he had heard a lecture early in his medical school career that he never forgot.

At this lecture, his class was told that it was possible to make a person immune to the disease of diphtheria by inoculation with a vaccine made from killed diphtheria bacteria. The professor then said that the only way a person could become immune to a virus was to actually suffer the disease because a killed vaccine would not work with a viral disease. Salk said, "I remember exactly where I was sitting, exactly how I felt at the time—as if a light went on. I said both statements can't be true."[4]

In 1939, when Salk worked with Thomas Francis, little was known about the workings of viruses. In 1898 a scientist named Martinus Beijernick discovered something that was much smaller than bacteria. He isolated the substance that was causing a disease in tobacco plants and called it a *virus*—which means "poisonous slime" in Latin.[5]

Today we know that viruses, such as the ones that cause polio, chicken pox, influenza, colds, and AIDS, cannot live or reproduce alone. They first have to invade a living cell and instruct that cell's reproductive system to make thousands more viral particles. Those particles are then capable of infecting new cells as the disease spreads.

When the immune system recognizes that something foreign is present in the body, it begins to work to eliminate the invaders. Key elements in this defense are proteins called antibodies. If the immune system succeeds and rids the body of the bacteria or virus, the patient recovers. When that person's immune system comes into future contact with the same invader, it quickly mounts a ready-made defense to attack and subdue the infection.

This ability of the body to recognize and repel previously encountered viruses and bacteria is called immunity. At the time that Jonas Salk studied with Dr. Francis, the science of immunology was just in its beginning stages.

Natural immunity is created when a person actually experiences and survives a disease such as polio or chicken pox. Scientists such as Francis also believed that immunity to infections could be created artificially. The trick was to develop vaccines in which the viruses or bacteria were killed or weakened enough so that they would not cause the illness in people being inoculated.

On the other hand, a vaccine had to have enough "power" left to fool the body into recognizing a foreign invader. Then antibodies to fight the virus could be rapidly produced in the bloodstream. When a vaccine causes antibodies to be produced, the inoculated person becomes immune to that particular infection, should natural exposure occur in the future.

The work that Jonas Salk did with Thomas Francis revolved around the manufacture and use of vaccines to prevent illness. Salk learned valuable theories and techniques during those two months of his senior year in 1939. He also developed a profound interest in the complex and fascinating world of the bacteriologist.

During his last year in medical school, Jonas found another profound interest—her name was Donna Lindsay. She was an attractive, intelligent student at the New York School of Social Work. A graduate of Smith College with a degree in psychology, Donna intended to help people less fortunate than herself by studying to become a social worker. The two spent what little free time they had together. Then on June 9, 1939—the day after Jonas Salk graduated from medical school—the couple was married.

4

Salk's First Work with Vaccines

New physicians were required to spend two years working in a hospital under the guidance of more experienced medical personnel before they could practice medicine on their own. As Salk waited to hear where he would be assigned for his internship, he continued to work in the laboratory of Dr. Francis. When Jonas finally received word that he would be an intern at Mount Sinai Hospital in New York City, he was very pleased. To be chosen for one of the twelve spaces available for student doctors at this respected institution was considered an honor.

At Mount Sinai Hospital the young and eager Dr. Salk worked well with his fellow interns. He also treated the patients under his care with understanding and sympathy. Salk was able to examine ill patients and correctly diagnose their diseases. In addition he showed a great deal of skill when performing surgery. Doctor Salk was admired and respected by both the patients and staff, and would likely have made a very good private physician. Yet in spite of his obvious clinical talents, Salk's main interest continued to revolve around the world of research.

The intern's exhausting schedule included long shifts and frequent weekend work—all for a salary of only $15 a month! In addition to his hospital duties, Salk wanted to spend time at home with his wife Donna. Doctor Salk didn't have very many extra hours in his life, but those that he could find were spent in the laboratory.

In 1942, at the end of his two-year internship, Jonas Salk began to look for a job in some area of research. After he was turned down for several positions in the New York region, he wrote a letter to his former employer. By then Dr. Thomas Francis had moved to the University of Michigan in Ann Arbor and was the head of the department of epidemiology. An epidemiologist tracks the location and pattern of diseases such as influenza or polio, trying to discover ways to stop the diseases from spreading.

The beginning of World War II made Francis's work very important. It was crucial to have an effective influenza vaccine that would prevent another epidemic of the virus similar to the one that claimed so many soldiers' lives during World War I. Francis had done work with live or weakened virus vaccines for some time. When injected into a person, a weakened or "attenuated" virus is not powerful enough to cause illness. But it is still able to alert the immune system to produce antibodies. Technically a virus cannot be called either "alive" or "dead." The slang terms "killed" and "live" are commonly used, though, to describe inactivated and attenuated virus vaccines.

A British scientist named Edward Jenner created the first successful vaccine in 1796. He saw that people who milked cows and were exposed to the disease of cowpox usually did not catch smallpox. Smallpox was a very serious viral illness that was fatal to as many as 40 percent of those who contracted it. Sometimes the disease blinded its victims or left them with terrible scars on their faces where the sores had been.

Jenner experimented with just one eight-year-old boy by scratching some material from a cowpox sore into the boy's arm. Later Jenner exposed the boy to the human smallpox virus, and no illness occurred. The antibodies that developed in the boy's blood as a result of the cowpox vaccine also protected him from smallpox.

This vaccine became widely used during the next 183 years. Later, in 1979, the World Health Organization (WHO) announced that the entire world was free of the once deadly disease of smallpox—thanks to Jenner's original work with cowpox.[1]

Francis believed that immunity to a disease could

also be possible by using a killed virus vaccine. In addition he felt that a killed vaccine would be much safer than a live one. The possibility existed that a live but weakened virus could suddenly become strong or virulent again, producing the illness that it was designed to prevent.

For reasons of safety, the military was interested only in a killed vaccine for the soldiers. The Armed Forces Epidemiological Board enlisted the help of Dr. Francis, who was already working with the influenza virus. Since he needed extra help in the laboratory, Francis offered Jonas Salk the opportunity to assist in the influenza work. Salk was eager to take the $40-a-week job. He and Donna moved to Ann Arbor, Michigan, in 1942.

As work in the laboratory progressed, a field trial to test the flu vaccine was scheduled. Frequent trips to a nearby army base were part of Dr. Salk's duties. He took medical histories from the servicemen. Then he injected the soldiers with the experimental vaccine that he helped to develop.

After a time he returned to interview the men about their reactions to the shots. He also collected information about the number of cases of influenza that had occurred on the base. With Salk's help, the trials were successfully completed and the data analyzed. The killed influenza virus vaccine was found to be effective and was widely used on U.S. soldiers during World War II.

Salk's life away from the laboratory was spent in an

old farmhouse that he and Donna rented. They planted a large vegetable garden and learned to cook on the wood-burning kitchen stove. A son, named Peter, was born to the young couple in 1944, and in 1947, son Darrell was born. A third boy, named Jonathan, would be born after the family left Michigan. Along with her role as a mother, Donna Salk was eager to pursue her career, and took a job as a social worker.

In addition to their work with influenza, Francis and Salk received funds from the National Foundation for Infantile Paralysis (NFIP) to study polio epidemics. The NFIP, later nicknamed the March of Dimes, was organized in 1938 by President Franklin D. Roosevelt, who was partially paralyzed by polio. The organization raised money to help victims of polio. It also supported research into the causes and possible prevention of the disease.

5

Franklin Roosevelt
and Polio

Franklin Roosevelt's introduction to polio took place in the summer of 1921. At that time the future President had taken a vacation from his law practice. He was with his wife and five small children at their summer home in Maine. One day Roosevelt began to feel sick, and thinking that he had a summer cold, went to bed to rest. His slight fever and headache soon got much worse, and before long he experienced severe pain in his neck and back. Only when his legs, arms, and back became paralyzed did the doctors decide that Roosevelt had polio.

Even though adults got polio, the disease that was originally called infantile paralysis most often struck the young. A thirty-nine-year-old man was not its usual victim, and Roosevelt's doctors did not even suspect polio at first. After the disease was correctly identified there was very little that could be done for the partially paralyzed man. Unfortunately there was no cure for polio once it infected a person, so Roosevelt could only rest in bed and hope that one day he would be able to move his arms and legs again.

After Franklin Roosevelt began to feel a little better, he made several visits to a resort in Georgia called Warm Springs. Although it was apparent that he would never walk again without the support of crutches and leg braces, he thought that exercise in the warm mineral water made his legs feel stronger and less stiff. Maybe a visit to the springs would help other polio victims also.

Because many polio patients' nerve cells are killed or damaged by the virus, incomplete messages are relayed to the muscles of the arms and legs. The limbs often become twisted into unnatural positions and are held there by painful spasms. Physical therapy in warm water to help loosen up the stiff muscles was a technique that became more popular as polio was better understood. Earlier methods of treatment had often not been as gentle.

At one time doctors believed that legs and arms that were twisted into strange positions by the disease simply needed to be straightened. A leg that was bent back at the knee would be forcibly stretched out and encased in a plaster cast to hold it straight. The patient suffered a

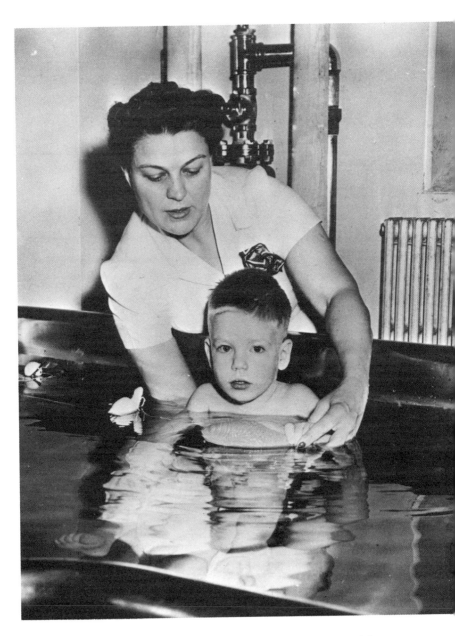

This boy is receiving physical therapy in warm water. The water therapy helped loosen stiff muscles that accompanied polio.

great deal of pain as the leg fought to return to its bent position.

In later years doctors realized that paralyzed bodies responded much better to less extreme treatment. Gentle exercise in heated water allowed the limbs to be moved gradually and the muscles to relax their unnatural spasms. Even before the therapy was widely used, Roosevelt knew that he felt better after a dip in the naturally heated water in Georgia. Consequently he, his law partner Basil O'Connor, and several supporters, bought the hotel at Warm Springs as well as the grounds around the resort.

A rehabilitation center was established there for polio patients. People partially paralyzed by the disease could visit, swim in the warm pools, and get some physical therapy. Most important, they could be with others like themselves and talk of their fears, frustrations, and hopes.

By the time that Franklin Roosevelt was elected as the thirty-second President of the United States in 1932, the rehabilitation center was in serious financial trouble. The Depression had taken its toll on people's incomes, and donations were not large enough to keep Warm Springs open. In an attempt to raise money to save the center, 6,000 Presidential Dances were held in communities all across America on Roosevelt's fifty-first birthday. Thousands of people attended and made contributions that eventually amounted to over one million dollars.

In a radio broadcast on the night of his birthday, Roosevelt said, "It is with a humble and thankful heart that I accept this tribute through me to the stricken ones of our great national family. I thank you but lack the words to tell you how deeply I appreciate what you have done and I bid you good night on what is to me the happiest birthday I have ever known."[1]

This was not the end of Roosevelt's involvement with polio. Before long the rehabilitation center was again in financial trouble. The recently formed NFIP launched a new campaign called the March of Dimes in 1938. The American people were asked to contribute any small amount of money that they could spare. They were told that even a dime was important in the war against polio.

The public responded to the idea with such enthusiasm that more than two and a half million dimes, or $250,000, poured into the White House during the next several weeks. Children raided their piggy banks and sent dimes that were sometimes carefully wrapped up in layers of sticky tape so that they wouldn't get lost. A few imaginative cooks even baked dimes into beautifully decorated cakes and mailed them to the President in Washington, D.C.

The dimes and larger contributions finally amounted to nearly two million dollars! The successful March of

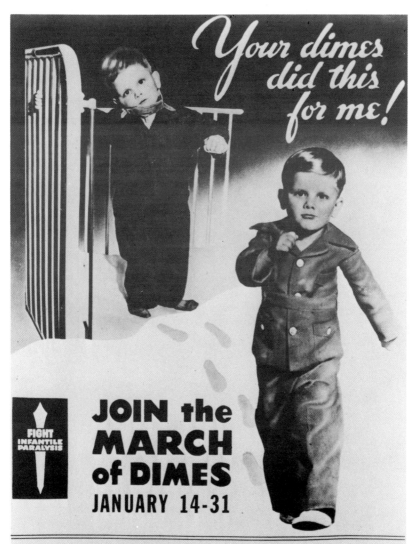

The March of Dimes campaign began in 1938. Over the years, posters such as this one were used to encourage people to donate whatever money they could spare to the cause.

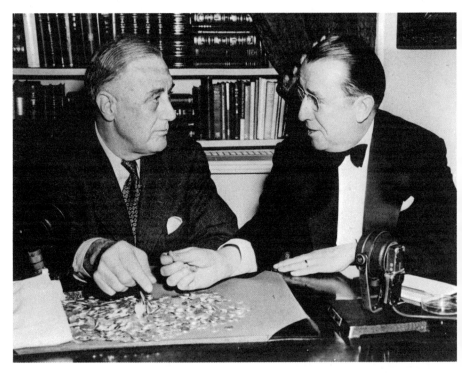

President Roosevelt met with Basil O'Connor, president of the NFIP, to count some of the many dimes received from the March of Dimes campaign.

Dimes campaign continued to be held annually to raise money for polio. This campaign money helped support the work that Francis and Salk were engaged in at the University of Michigan.

Although Jonas Salk enjoyed his work with Dr. Francis and learned a great deal from the talented man, he wanted to be the director of his own laboratory. Then he would be able to do the research that most interested him—and do it in his own way. After five years at the University of Michigan, an opportunity arose for Salk to do just that.

6

The University
of Pittsburgh

The medical school at the University of Pittsburgh was not an especially impressive place when Jonas Salk first arrived there in 1947. Most of the faculty members were doctors from town who taught part-time at the facility, and no important research was being conducted. The administrators wanted to change the image of their school.

Salk was invited to join the university's staff as a Research Professor of Bacteriology and operate his own virus research laboratory. Salk's colleagues in Michigan tried to persuade him to refuse the offer. They argued that his reputation could only be diminished by working at such a (then) mediocre institution. Salk, on the other hand, was frustrated and wanted to be independent. He decided to accept the offer extended by the University of

Pittsburgh. In 1947 he moved his wife and two young sons to a suburb of Pittsburgh that was eighteen miles from the university.

In reality Salk's position was even less than he had been led to expect. He was an Associate Professor of Bacteriology, and every request that he made had to be approved by a superior. His laboratory turned out to be a 40 x 40 foot space in the basement of the Municipal Hospital, which was located across the street from the medical school. Maybe his new job would prove to be a mistake, just as his friends predicted.

Despite the disappointments Salk arranged his small laboratory and began work on an improved influenza vaccine. His tiny quarters didn't prevent him from developing a new version of the influenza vaccine that doubled the period of immunity for those who got the shots.

In 1948, three years after President Franklin Roosevelt died from a cerebral hemorrhage, the NFIP decided to sponsor a series of studies designed to find out how many different types of polio virus existed. Before a vaccine could be developed, more had to be learned about the disease. Four laboratories located at the Universities of Pittsburgh, Utah, Kansas, and Southern California were asked to perform the same experiments simultaneously and then compare their results.

Henry Weaver, NFIP Research Director, offered

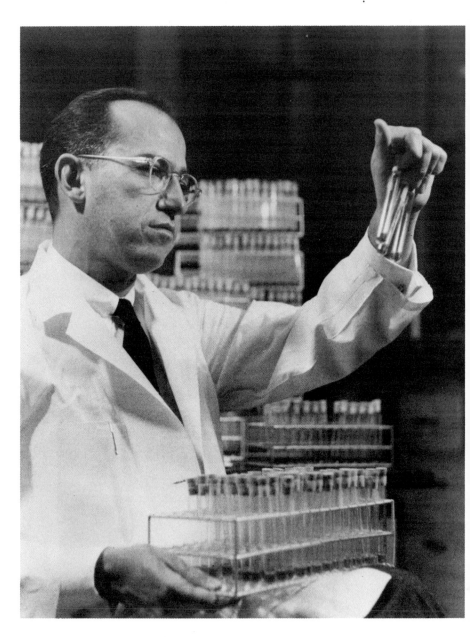

Dr. Salk in his University of Pittsburgh laboratory. His early work focused on finding an improved influenza vaccine.

Dr. Salk and the University of Pittsburgh a $200,000 grant to participate in the virus typing or classification program. In spite of the fact that much of the work would be tedious and repetitious, Salk agreed to be a part of the project. He saw it as an opportunity to finally be in charge of his own research program and have a reliable source of funds.

There were many diseases such as influenza that infected and killed thousands more people than polio did, but a case of influenza was not usually as dramatic. It was hard to tell who had been a victim of the influenza virus because once the patient recovered, there were no lasting effects. Polio, on the other hand, left visible evidence of its damage in the form of atrophied arms and legs, curved spines, and paralyzed bodies, which very often belonged to young children.

The early symptoms of polio were like those of many other illnesses: a sore throat, upset stomach, headache, and a slight fever. Most of the people who had the disease never got very sick and recovered from the infection in a few days. However, in some the fever rose, and the neck and back became painful and stiff.

As the virus attacked the central nervous system, lines of communication between the brain and the muscles were damaged or destroyed. When the muscles no longer received messages from the brain, they stopped moving and became paralyzed. Sometimes the motor nerve cells were only damaged and recovered so that the paralysis was temporary. However, if the cells were destroyed they could not regenerate, and the affected muscles remained useless forever.[1]

A visit to the children's polio ward in any hospital was all that it took to be convinced of the desperate need for a vaccine to stop the epidemics. Tired nurses hurried back and forth to huge vats of boiling water that were full of steaming wool blankets. The heavy blankets were wrung out and placed over painful arms and legs. This moist heat gradually relaxed the muscle spasms and allowed some children to sleep for short periods of time—in spite of the continuous noise around them.[2]

Added to the sounds of human suffering were the mechanical hisses from "iron lungs." These large metal cylinders contained the critically ill patients who had bulbar polio. This was the most serious form of polio and involved an area of the lower brain called the bulb.

In bulbar polio, the nerve cells in the brain stem that automatically control breathing were damaged or destroyed by the virus so that the patient could no longer breathe naturally. Twenty-four-hour-a-day assistance from the iron lung was necessary to keep the paralyzed victim alive.

An electric motor pumped air into the metal tube. Inside, added pressure on the patient's body caused the chest to compress so that air was forced out of the lungs through the nose and mouth. As air was let out of the chamber, pressure decreased and allowed the chest to rise

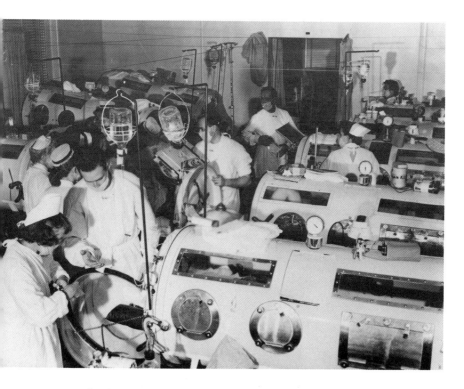

Critically ill polio patients were placed in "iron lungs," which were machines that helped them breathe.

and the lungs to expand and fill with air. A snug rubber collar fit around the patient's neck to create a seal that kept the air inside the chamber.

Twice a day the bulbar polio patients were briefly put onto portable breathing machines so that they could be rolled out of their hot metal beds and bathed. The portable devices wrapped around the front of the upper body and pushed in and out on the chest. As the machine pushed down on the chest, air was expelled from the lungs. Then, as the pressure was released, the lungs expanded and air was drawn in. This method was less satisfactory than the iron lung because constant motion on the chest produced skin irritation and soreness to the underlying tissues.

Rocking beds were used to stimulate those whose breathing ability was damaged but not totally destroyed. The electric beds rocked up and down like a seesaw. As the head of the bed went down, the patient's head also descended while the feet went up. Thus the internal organs fell forward, pressing on the lungs and helping to push the air out of them.

When the head of the bed came back up, the patient's head also rose. Then the organs fell back into place and the pressure was taken off of the lungs so that they could fill with air. The rocking beds were hot exhausting work for their occupants. Many struggling patients often felt like they would not be able to get their next breath.[3]

Most of the polio epidemics of the 1940s and 1950s occurred during the summer months. Hot temperatures in the wards were a serious problem that affected staff members as well as patients. Heat from the vats of boiling water, hot blankets, and constantly running electric motors added to the problem. Unfortunately air conditioning was not yet widely available in the United States.

Clothing and bed linen needed to be changed often, and small feverish bodies had to be kept clean with frequent sponge baths. Nurses worked until they were exhausted, stopping for only a brief rest before returning to duty. Some of the older children who were feeling better were able to play games with each other or read stories to the younger patients, and thus, help the overworked staff members.

Television was not yet in general use but radio programs provided some escape from the long hours of sickness and boredom. Baseball games, especially the World Series, were followed closely by many of those who could do little except lie quietly in bed.

Some parents were allowed into the wards to serve as volunteers. All of them had to be dressed from head to foot in sterile white garments that included face masks. No one was really sure just how polio was transmitted, and every precaution was taken to prevent the spread of the disease. All eating utensils, linens, and instruments

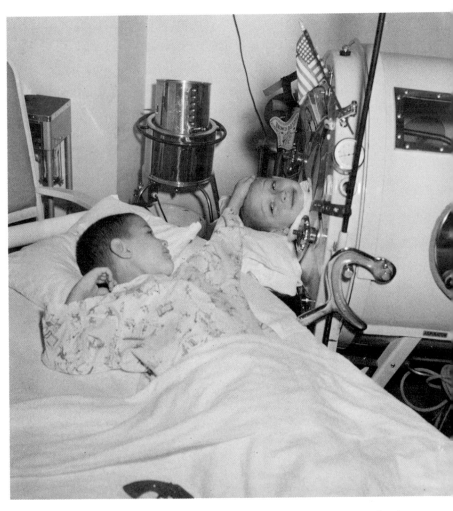

These twin brothers both suffered from polio and were hospitalized in the same room. Every year seemed to bring an increasing number of new polio cases.

from the polio wards had to be sterilized separately from those used in the rest of the hospital.[4]

At Municipal Hospital in Pittsburgh the wards were filled with an ever-increasing number of polio patients. Even though polio most often targeted the very young, adults also became victims of the disease. Infected mothers and fathers lay helpless in bed, no longer able to provide for their families as they fought to get well. Occasionally a healthy baby was even born in an iron lung to a paralyzed mother who was unable to breathe normally on her own.

Doctor Salk had ample opportunity to see firsthand the ravages of the disease. He liked children and worried about the health of his own young sons. To see a small helpless child suffering in pain or encased in an iron lung was a painful sight. A quick walk through the hospital made it clear that a better understanding of the polio virus was badly needed.

In time it was learned that the polio virus entered the body through the nose or mouth and traveled to the intestines. In a small percentage of infected people, the virus then passed into the bloodstream and continued on to the central nervous system—especially the motor nerve cells of the spinal cord. Ironically polio was an epidemic problem in countries where there was a high standard of living and good sanitary conditions.

In poor countries that did not have adequate sewage treatment facilities and a clean water supply, most children were exposed to the virus very early in life. At that age they still had the partial immunity to infections that babies are born with. Infants who were infected with polio almost always had only a mild illness. From that time on there were antibodies in their blood that protected them from the disease in later years.[5]

In clean and sanitary environments, early childhood contact with the polio virus was uncommon. Antibodies, therefore, did not exist in the blood of most children and many adults. When polio struck those past infancy, the effects of the disease could be very serious.

7

Virus Typing

Before Jonas Salk could start to work on the NFIP's polio virus typing program, he had to design a laboratory that was large enough to handle the increased amount of work. Additional staff was also needed to run the thousands of experiments that would be conducted. Catalogs and drawings littered the small basement space that Salk used for his research projects at the University of Pittsburgh.

Rooms to house cages had to be built for the laboratory animals that would be used in the experiments. Temperature-controlled storage areas were also necessary because some materials would have to be kept warm and others cool in refrigerators. The NFIP pledged to support the scientific work with a $200,000 grant, but Salk had to find another source of funds for the renovations and equipment. The foundation wouldn't pay for construction costs.

Rather than resent all of the time he spent designing storage spaces, ordering supplies, and searching for funds, Salk seemed to enjoy getting his new laboratory in order. His original tiny basement room would eventually grow into a laboratory that occupied several unused floors of the Municipal Hospital building and provided employment for dozens of people.

When the construction was finally finished and extra staff hired, the time had finally arrived to begin the actual job of virus typing. The scientific community generally believed that three types of polio virus existed and that each type had many different strains. Salk's laboratory, along with the three others, would test this theory.

Each facility would classify samples from more than 100 unidentified polio strains that had been isolated from patients who had been infected with the disease. At the end of the three-year project, the data would be compared to see if all four testing laboratories arrived at the same conclusions.

In order to classify each of the 100-plus viruses, a standard procedure was to be followed. Monkeys were used in the experiments because they were the only animals that could be effectively infected with the polio virus. The process began when a group of monkeys was infected with an already identified polio virus such as

Type I. The animals then got sick and either recovered or died. Those that recovered had antibodies in their blood for the Type I polio virus and should be immune to it in the future.

These recently recovered monkeys were then given an untyped polio virus from the 100-plus samples. If they remained well, the unidentified virus was probably also Type I. If the monkeys got sick again, the virus was assumed to be Type II or III since the animal's blood would not have antibodies to fight either of those types. As soon as one of the samples was identified, the procedure was repeated for the next sample until all of the more than 100 viruses were typed.[1]

The method seemed clear-cut, but there were many things that could go wrong. One monkey might be naturally more resistant to disease than another. Or a particular batch of virus might be just a little more or less potent and not work in exactly the same manner as the preceding batch.

A constant supply of monkeys was needed for the work, and since the animals were not bred in captivity, they had to be captured in the wild. For the most commonly used rhesus monkeys, the journey began in India where the animals were coaxed out of the trees and put into bamboo cages. The cages were then carried out of the jungle to be put aboard a train for a ride to the nearest airport.

Once at the airport, the longest part of the journey

began—the nearly 8,000-mile trip to New York City. A full-time attendant remained with the monkeys to see that they received food and water three times a day. After the animals arrived in the United States, they were shipped to the various sites where polio research was being conducted.

Since four laboratories were working on the virus typing programs simultaneously, thousands of animals were needed. After their long journey, the monkeys who arrived at the universities needed extra attention to adjust to their new surroundings. Frequently the laboratories did not have enough staff members to adequately handle the new arrivals.

The difficulties became so great that the NFIP decided to set up a "monkey holding" facility in South Carolina. After it opened, the primates were shipped directly to this facility and allowed to rest and recover from their journey. The monkeys that arrived at Okatie Farms spent an average of three weeks there.[2]

Once at Salk's laboratory, the monkeys needed a regular attendant to take care of them. Their cages had to be cleaned often, and so did the animals themselves. The monkeys made the job more difficult when they spread food and feces around their cages. Sometimes the animals threw a handful of whatever was available at their visitors! Those who worked in adjoining parts of the building occasionally complained about the noise and smells coming from the monkey quarters.

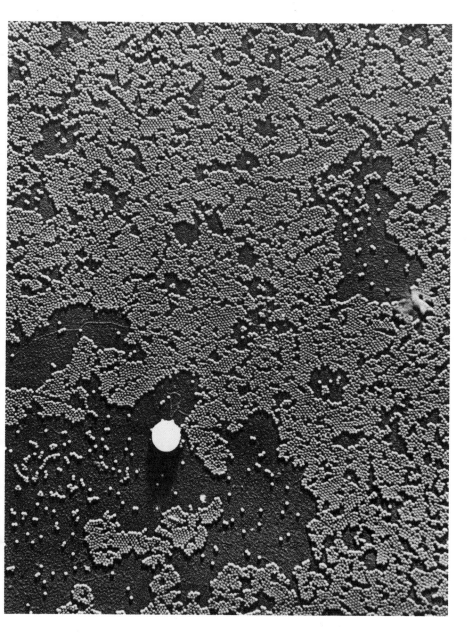

The polio virus greatly magnified. The large white dot is a marker.
Salk worked to identify the three types of this virus.

In spite of the mess though, the patients and hospital staff liked to visit the monkeys. They enjoyed watching the monkeys' entertaining and silly behavior as they chattered and played with each other. Occasionally, however, visitors had to dodge a "monkey missile" that was launched from one of the cages.

Because the monkeys could sometimes seem almost human, staff members often became attached to certain ones. They frequently felt sad because so many had to be sacrificed during the experiments. But a quick walk through the polio ward would help to convince the scientists that the monkeys were a regrettable but necessary tragedy in the war against polio.

Seeing patients in pain and hearing iron lungs wheezing life into paralyzed bodies made the scientists eager to get back to their work in the lab. Unfortunately the repetitious experiments took so many animals and so much time. The disease might strike thousands more during the years that it would take to find answers to the polio problem.

Before long Dr. Salk devised a way to make the virus typing faster and easier. Using his method, he gave a monkey a large dose of untyped polio virus. After the animal recovered from the illness, some of its blood was mixed into test tubes that contained samples of each of the three known types of polio viruses.

The material in the test tubes was then studied to see if the antibodies in the monkey's blood had neutralized the Type I, II, or III polio virus. When the neutralized sample was identified, the unknown virus was assumed to be of the same type. Salk's method used far fewer laboratory animals and took much less time to complete.[3]

When Salk approached his fellow researchers and the NFIP with a request to use his new virus typing technique, he was turned down. He reminded them that both time and many animals could be saved, but the NFIP officers replied that all four laboratories had to conduct the same tests in exactly the same manner or the results would not be valid. He did succeed in getting approval to conduct the experiments his way in addition to the approved way. In effect that would make his data twice as reliable because results from the two types of experiments could be compared in his own laboratory.

By the summer of 1950, the same year that their third son, Jonathan, was born to Jonas and Donna, Dr. Salk was ready to begin work on a polio vaccine. The biggest problem that Salk encountered in the production of a vaccine was the huge amount of virus that would be needed to conduct the experiments. Viruses would not grow in a glass dish full of culture medium as bacteria did. Viruses could only be grown within living cells, and polio grew only in human or monkey cells.

Many scientists had tried to grow the virus outside of a living body. In 1936 Dr. Albert Sabin succeeded in growing polio virus in test tubes of human tissue taken from the central nervous system. He was not able to grow it in any other kind of tissue and assumed that none of the polio virus strains would grow in anything except nervous tissue.

Since past experience showed that people often had severe and sometimes fatal reactions to vaccines that were grown in nervous tissue, this method of vaccine production could not be safely used. At that time Sabin did not test any other strains of the virus to see if they would grow in different kinds of tissue.

It was not until 1949 that another attempt was made to grow polio virus in non-nervous tissue. This time the strain that was used did multiply. The successful attempt by Dr. John Enders and his assistants, Dr. Frederick Robbins and Dr. Thomas Weller, paved the way for the creation of a vaccine. Their discovery meant that polio virus could now be grown in large amounts without the danger of contamination by nervous tissue.

Before the Nobel-Prize-winning discovery, monkeys were used as "factories" to produce the virus. Many monkeys were needed to supply the laboratory with only a small amount of polio virus. After Enders's discovery, large quantities of the virus could be grown in test tubes of non-nervous monkey tissue collected from only a few animals.

Salk was eager to try this new technique. He got some starter cultures from Enders and learned how to grow the virus using monkey kidney tissue. The tissue

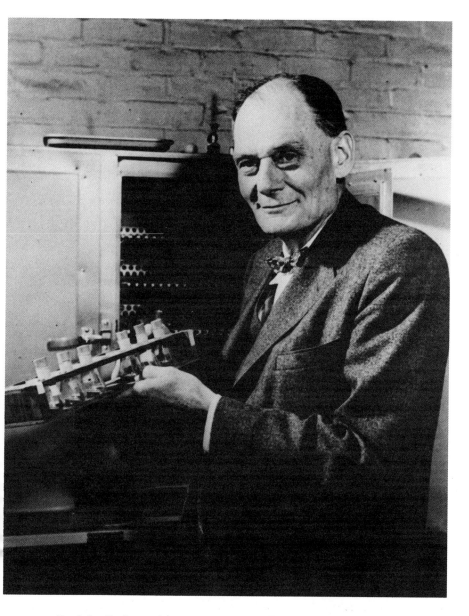

Dr. John Enders and his assistants successfully grew the polio virus in non-nervous tissue. His work paved the way for the creation of a polio vaccine.

was cut into tiny pieces and put into bottles of a solution that encouraged it to continue to grow—just as if it were still living. After about six days, live polio virus was added to the mixture and allowed to multiply for a few days until it reached the right concentration. Diluted formaldehyde, called formalin, was then added to the mixture to inactivate the virus but not destroy it completely.[4]

It took months of experiments to discover exactly the right way to grow the cultures and at what temperature the kidney cells and viruses multiplied best. In addition Salk and his team had to learn how much formalin was needed to kill the virus. Every single virus had to be dead or the vaccine would be capable of causing polio in those who were inoculated.

To determine if any live virus remained, a sample was taken from every batch of vaccine that was produced. It was added to a solution that contained monkey kidney tissue. Several days later the kidney cells were examined under a microscope to see if there was any viral damage.

Live monkeys were also used to test the vaccine's safety. Some were given shots of the solution and were then watched carefully for any symptoms of polio. Dr. Salk was extremely careful to make sure that no live viruses slipped into his vaccine.[5]

In September 1951 an international conference on polio was held in Denmark, and Dr. Jonas Salk was

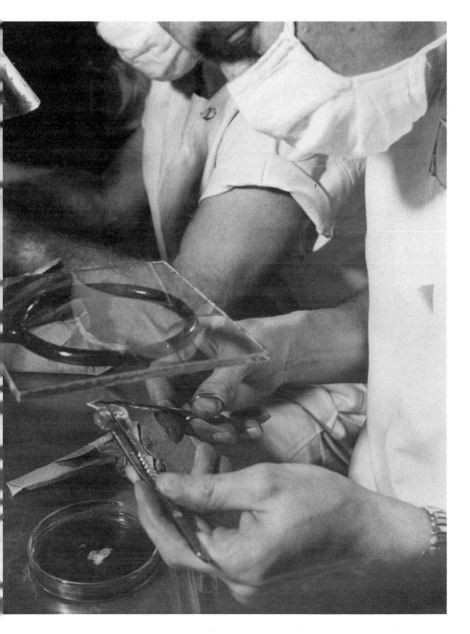

Salk used monkey kidney tissues to grow the polio virus. Here, a lab worker cuts the tissue into tiny pieces.

asked to give a speech about the virus typing program. He reported on his experiments and said that there were almost certainly only three types of polio virus. There were many different strains of the disease-causing virus, but they all fit into the three main categories. A vaccine that contained a representative strain from each of the three types would protect people against all kinds of polio.

During the cruise back home from Denmark Jonas Salk and Basil O'Connor, president of the NFIP, got to know each other better. They had worked together in the past, but never found the time for any long conversations. Many idle hours at sea gave the men an opportunity to talk not only about polio but about themselves as well. They got along very well and developed a great respect for each other. O'Connor's interest in Salk would play a big part in the young scientist's future.

8

Polio Vaccine

By 1952 Salk's virus typing program was finished and his vaccine work had progressed to the point that he was ready to begin human tests. The very first people to test a new vaccine always take a calculated risk. Any previously untested product is capable of producing serious illness or even death. Salk had enough confidence in his vaccine to give it to himself first and then to those who worked with him. Thirty years later when he was asked about those early injections he said, "You wouldn't do unto others that which you wouldn't do unto yourself."[1] No negative reactions were observed in Salk or his inoculated laboratory assistants.

All of Salk's early inoculation work was done in secret. If the public thought that there were a vaccine available, even if it were only experimental, they might demand that it be used before proper testing could take place. Public anxiety was fueled by the fact that one of the worst polio epidemics in history was raging across the country in 1952. Nearly 60,000 people were victims of the crippling disease during that year.[2]

Salk needed time to administer and observe the results of his vaccine to make sure that it was safe and effective. Therefore, when the time arrived to inoculate volunteers, the work was done in strict confidence.

Salk went to the Watson Home for Crippled Children for one of his early tests. The children who lived at the beautiful country estate were already disabled by polio. Even though a vaccine would arrive too late to help them, many volunteered to be test subjects in the hope that they could help prevent others from getting the disease in the future.

To conduct the experiment, Salk had to find out which type of polio virus had infected each child. He did that by taking samples of the children's blood back to his laboratory for antibody analysis. If he found that a patient had been infected by a Type I virus, he then gave that child a Type I vaccine. Type I antibodies would already be in the blood from the original infection, and he wanted to see if the vaccine would increase the antibody levels in the victim's blood. He used the same procedure with Types II and III polio patients.

Once the shots were given, Dr. Salk had to wait to see what the results would be. During the summer months of 1952 he made many trips to the Watson Home to check on the status of the patients. The children enjoyed his visits because he remembered their names and listened to the stories they told to him about their friends and families at home.

When all of the Watson Home results were analyzed, it was apparent that the vaccine caused the children's systems to boost production of antibodies higher than those from the original infection. Also none of the forty-five children who participated in the study got sick or experienced any bad reactions from the inoculations. During the next several months after the successful trial, Salk went on to test his vaccine on several more small groups in the Pittsburgh area.

Early in 1953 a conference was held by the NFIP Immunization Committee. During one of the meetings Jonas Salk reported on his "secret" vaccine tests and proposed that a larger trial was needed. Doctor Albert Sabin, a member of the committee and a vocal critic, thought that Salk was moving much too fast. Sabin believed that many more years of careful study were needed before a massive field trial could be conducted.

Following the meeting, details of the discussions were reported in a medical journal. Before long, newspapers and magazines began to run stories about the possibility of a polio vaccine in the near future. The news spread quickly and people demanded to know more. If a vaccine was available why wasn't it being used?

To answer some of the questions, Jonas Salk spoke to the American people on March 26, 1953, in a radio program called "The Scientist Speaks for Himself." He talked about the vaccine and how it worked, and said that it would be dangerous to rush it into production. The vaccine needed to be tested very carefully before it could be used for the general public. Salk also reminded his listeners that contributions to the NFIP were necessary to keep polio research going. From that time on, everything that Dr. Salk did was closely watched and reported. America was more than ready for a polio vaccine.

By the spring of 1953 Salk had developed a vaccine that included representative strains of all three types of the polio virus. He took enough of the material home for shots for himself, his wife Donna, and their three sons. At that time Peter was nine; Darrell, six; and Jonathan, only three. Doctor Salk was confident that the vaccine was not dangerous. He did not yet know how long it would provide immunity to those who were inoculated. The important task was to get some protection for his family and the rest of the country as quickly as possible.

During the next few months Salk inoculated several thousand children and adults who lived in the Pittsburgh area. When no bad reactions were observed from the vaccine he felt that it was time to move on to a much larger test. NFIP president Basil O'Connor created a Vaccine Advisory Committee to study the possibility of a

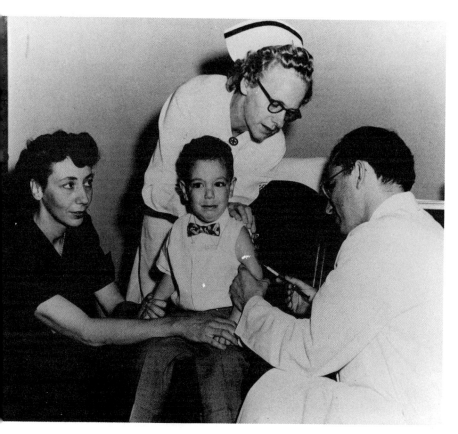

Salk had such confidence in his vaccine that he even tested it on his own three sons. Here, he administers the vaccine to his youngest son, Jonathan.

field trial. O'Connor was ready to use the March of Dimes money to support Salk and a nationwide test of the vaccine.

Doctor Albert Sabin once again voiced strong objections to a large field trial. He and several other virologists believed that a small number of people needed to be inoculated and then studied for several years to test the safety of the vaccine. He also felt that Salk's inactivated vaccine would only offer short-term immunity and that frequent booster shots would be needed to make the vaccine effective. Sabin was convinced that the only way to obtain lasting immunity to polio was with a "live" virus vaccine.

The debate continued until Basil O'Connor stepped in and made the decision to proceed with a field trial. O'Connor's thirty-year-old daughter, Bettyann, had become a victim of polio in 1950. She was the mother of five small children when she was paralyzed.

All O'Connor could see was a future filled with more and more polio patients similar to Bettyann. He had confidence in Jonas Salk and believed that the time had come to put Salk's vaccine to the test. None of the people who had been vaccinated at the Watson Home or in the Pittsburgh area had shown any ill effects from the shots.

Salk was also confident of the vaccine, but knew that his small laboratory could not produce enough of it to conduct a large trial. Other laboratories would have to be enlisted to manufacture the vaccine according to

Salk's specifications, and this fact caused concern. Salk's work was very carefully controlled, and the vaccine was checked again and again for any signs of live virus. He wondered if another laboratory would be as cautious.

To ease Salk's fears it was agreed that each batch of vaccine produced would be examined by the company making it, by the National Institutes of Health, and by Salk's laboratory. For success to occur it was crucial that no live virus remain. If anyone got polio from a bad batch of vaccine, the entire test program might fail.

As the field trial neared, the two laboratories that were involved in vaccine production did, indeed, experience problems. An infectious virus appeared in several of the samples produced outside of Salk's laboratory. His procedure was carefully reviewed and the other labs were directed to follow the steps exactly. Eventually vaccines free from any traces of infectious polio virus were produced in enough quantity to proceed with the test.

Salk was constantly busy during the days before the field trial. The news media hounded him for details about the vaccine. He was featured in several magazine articles and newspaper stories. Many of Salk's peers in the scientific community criticized him for participating in all of the publicity. Sabin once again took the opportunity to say that the field trials were premature. Salk's workdays got longer and longer as details about how the trial would be run were reviewed.

In order to make the field trial as scientifically rigorous as possible, the NFIP and Jonas Salk decided to conduct both observed control and double blind studies. In the observed control study, some children would be given an actual polio vaccination. Others in the same age group would not be given the vaccine at all, but their health patterns would be studied during the weeks of the trial. A comparison of the two groups could then be made to determine if the children who were vaccinated had any symptoms or illnesses that were not observed in the unvaccinated group.

In the double blind study, a certain number of children would receive an actual polio vaccination. An additional number would get a shot that looked exactly like a polio vaccine but contained only an inert substance such as colored water. No one would know the difference between the two, not even the doctors who administered the inoculations. This procedure would prevent any personal bias from influencing the evaluations.

Only after all of the vaccines were given and the blood tests and other data were gathered would the two groups be identified. Their statistics could then be compared to see if the vaccinated group fared any better than the group given the dummy vaccine, also known as a placebo.

A double blind study required that a large number of records be kept and that the vaccine versus placebo group assignments be secret. A special person was needed to compile and interpret the mountains of data that would result from the two types of studies to be used during the field trial.

Salk's former employer, Dr. Thomas Francis, was approached about the job. He agreed to do the evaluation at the University of Michigan only if he could make the rules. Francis said that none of the results would be made public until all of the reports had been collected and analyzed by his team. The process would probably take up to a year to complete, and during that time not even Jonas Salk would know the results of the field trial.

With the laboratories geared up to produce the vaccine and the evaluation team selected, the actual mechanics of the huge experiment had to be worked out. Volunteers had always been an important part of the success of the NFIP and they would play a large role in the field trial.

For years parents and other volunteers had conducted door-to-door fund-raising campaigns to support the March of Dimes. Each city and town in America already had a support group in place that was ready to help again. They just needed to be told what to do and how to do it. These people were eager to participate, especially if their help might mean an end to polio.

9

Field Trial

The field trial of 1954 would involve nearly two million children in forty-four states. An army of doctors, nurses, and volunteers was needed to get the program underway. Medium-sized communities that had been hard hit by polio in the past were selected as test sites. Children who were between the ages of five and eight years old seemed to be the most common victims of polio so first-, second-, and third-graders were chosen to be immunized.[1]

Elementary schools were designated as vaccination centers since the children would already be there. Using simple stories and filmstrips, teachers taught their students about the polio vaccine. The children were told that they would be taking part in a very important study and were "Polio Pioneers." Their fear of shots was often replaced by pride when the young students realized that they would be involved in a historical program.

The NFIP distributed booklets that explained the field trial and tried to answer questions about the safety of the vaccine. Permission slips were sent home with the target students. The forms were worded so that parents had to request that their children be allowed to be a part of the program. Instead of being afraid of the vaccine, parents were anxious for anything that might protect their sons and daughters from polio. They only wished that other family members could also receive the vaccine.[2]

With thousands of volunteers in place and the vaccination centers set up, the day finally arrived to begin the field trial. Boxes of needles, small bandages, and lollipops were stacked in designated areas of the schools where the shots would be given. Vials of pink liquid that were either the actual polio vaccine or a colored-water placebo were ready for injection. The students appeared to be excited and a little nervous as they lined up to follow their teachers to the vaccination centers.

Photographers were everywhere, ready to capture the smiles and tears of the first Polio Pioneers as they bravely marched down the hallways. Some of the children seemed worried that the shots would hurt and a few cried softly. But most of the pioneers were proud to be a part of the chosen group. They had received special treatment, lots of extra attention, and were missing regular classes to take part in the experiment.

On April 26, 1954, a boy named Randy Kerr who lived in McLean, Virginia, became the first child to be officially vaccinated in the field trial. Thousands followed as the program moved along smoothly at most of the immunization sites. A few problems occurred when the actual vaccine and the placebo were mixed up and the test reports for those cases had to be thrown away.

On several occasions an inoculation center ran out of vaccine and had to rush in a new supply while the volunteers anxiously waited. And in Montgomery, Alabama, the African-American children who agreed to be Polio Pioneers had to get their shots outside. (In Alabama in 1954, black children were not allowed to enter the buildings where white children went to school.)[3]

On the whole, the field trial was amazingly successful, thanks to the dedication of the volunteers. Parents, doctors, nurses, and school personnel gave freely of their time to see that the vaccine received a fair test. This immense effort was willingly accomplished by adults who did not ever want to see another child suffer with polio.

Participants in the test numbered 1,830,000 children, with 441,131 receiving the actual polio vaccine in three separate shots during a period of five weeks. An

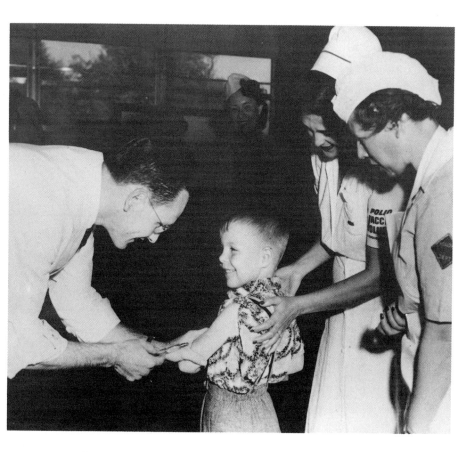

Randy Kerr of McLean, Virginia was officially the first child vaccinated with the polio vaccine in the field trial of 1954.

additional 201,229 children got three shots of dummy vaccine. The remaining children, who were only observed so that their health data could be compared with the ones who were vaccinated, numbered 1,063,951. Blood samples were taken from 2 percent of the children before the inoculations, and again after the shots were given.[4]

Some of the children didn't return for the full series of shots, and others were disqualified from the trial for a variety of reasons. When the numbers were tallied, they showed that 96 percent of the children who started the test program received all three shots. A few had mild reactions to the vaccination that included a slight headache, a little fever, and some soreness where the shot was given. But no one suffered a serious reaction as a result of the polio vaccine.

By the end of June all of the injections had been given and the field trial was over. Now it was time for Dr. Thomas Francis and his team of evaluators to sift through the mountains of reports and draw their conclusions. Stacks of medical records from all over the country arrived at the Vaccine Evaluation Center in Michigan.

Doctor Salk did not participate in the evaluation process and did not see any of the reports, even though he was very anxious to learn about the results of the program. The staff at the Evaluation Center had no prior connection to the field trial. Doctor Francis did not

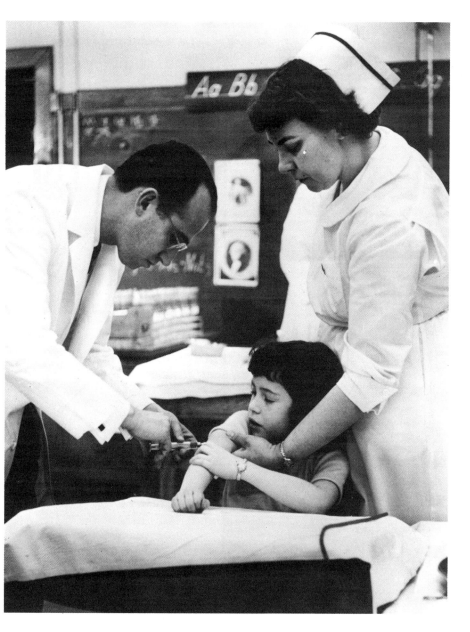

Dr. Salk administers the vaccine to a school girl during the field trial. Overall, 1,830,000 children participated in the test.

want hopes and expectations to color the outcome in any way and he demanded total secrecy until all of the results were analyzed.

Doctor Salk returned to his laboratory and resumed work on the polio vaccine. He wanted to make it even better than the one that was used in the field trial. Through experimentation he discovered that if the shots were spaced farther apart the vaccine could be even more effective.

During the field trial all three shots were given within a space of five weeks. Additional studies showed that shots one and two should be given during a four-week period. Then, if the third shot was not given for seven months, the body produced more polio antibodies and immunity to the disease lasted longer. Salk continued to work on the vaccine during the nine months that it took the evaluation team to compile its results.[5]

10

Vaccine Licensed

Finally on April 12, 1955, the entire nation and Dr. Salk himself heard the good news. Doctor Francis reported that the vaccine was 90 percent effective against the most serious Types II and III viruses and 70 percent effective against Type I. In addition the vaccine was considered safe because no serious reactions were observed among the Polio Pioneers and no cases of polio occurred as a result of the shots.

Within seven hours of the announcement, the government granted licenses to six large drug companies to manufacture the vaccine. Parke, Davis & Company; Cutter Laboratories; Wyeth Laboratories; Pitman-Moore Company; Sharp & Dohme; and Eli Lilly had already started to produce supplies of the vaccine in hopes that the trial results would be favorable. They would now be able to begin shipping the pink liquid almost immediately.[1]

Thousands of Americans called their doctors to ask when the shots would be available. Confusion followed in the first few days because no system was yet in place to distribute the vaccine. President Dwight Eisenhower requested that Oveta Culp Hobby—the Secretary of Health, Education, and Welfare—devise a plan that could be used to get the vaccine out into the hands of the doctors who would administer it.

As plans to distribute the vaccine were formulated, the Salk family was learning how to deal with instant fame. They became virtual prisoners in the University of Michigan guest house where they were staying. Photographers and reporters swarmed over the grounds around the house. They couldn't seem to get enough pictures and stories about Dr. Salk and his amazing achievement.

The telephone rarely stopped ringing as people called to offer their congratulations and thanks. Envelopes arrived with checks and cash, which Salk put into a fund that was to be used for more research. Peter, Darrell, and Jonathan quickly grew tired of wearing their good clothes. The Salk children wanted to go home where they could play outside and get dirty without a photographer around to snap their pictures.

After nearly a week in Michigan, the family was finally able to return to Pittsburgh. Things were not

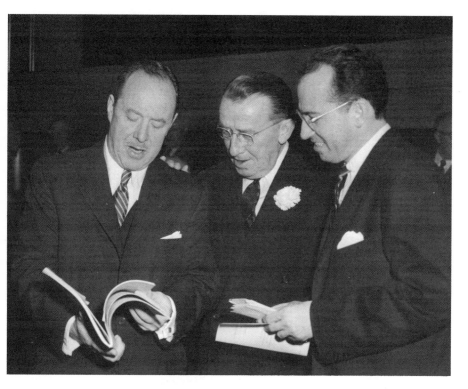

Dr. Salk (right) meets with Dr. Thomas Francis and Basil O'Connor after the news was announced that the polio vaccine was effective.

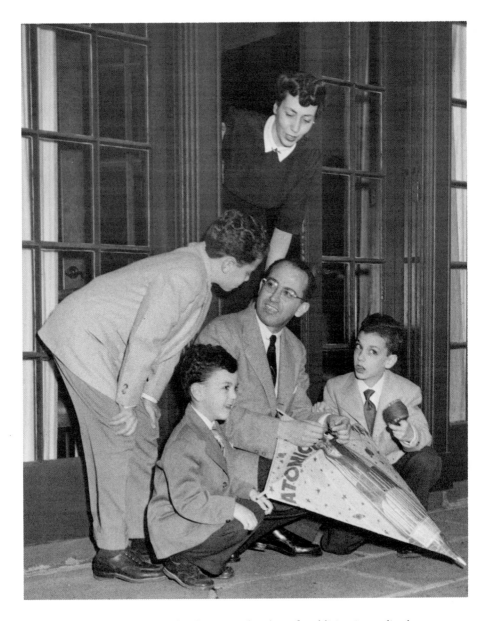

Dr. Salk and his family received a lot of publicity immediately following the announcement. Here, Salk poses with his wife, Donna, and three sons, Peter (age eleven), Jonathan (age five), and Darrell (age eight).

much better at home, for the public continued to shower Dr. Salk with their adulation. All across the country he was asked to give speeches to talk about the wonderful new vaccine. Someone even wanted to sell pajamas for children that had the words "Thank You, Dr. Salk" printed across the front. He agreed to give many of the speeches, but declined the offer to be immortalized on sleepwear.

While Jonas Salk was dealing with all of the attention—which included a trip to Washington, D.C., to receive a citation from President Eisenhower—the NFIP was trying to decide just who would get the vaccine. Everyone wanted it, but there was not enough available yet to inoculate the whole country. A plan was finally developed that provided free vaccinations to 7,000,000 children in the first, second, and third grades.

Also the Polio Pioneers who served as observed controls and the ones who received the dummy vaccinations would not have to pay for the inoculations. The rest of the pioneers who got the real vaccine would be given one booster shot because Salk determined that their original three shots were probably given too close together.[2]

President Eisenhower announced that knowledge of how to produce the vaccine would be shared with nations across the world so that they, too, could begin a vaccination program. Jonas Salk did not hold a patent on the vaccine because he developed it for the NFIP,

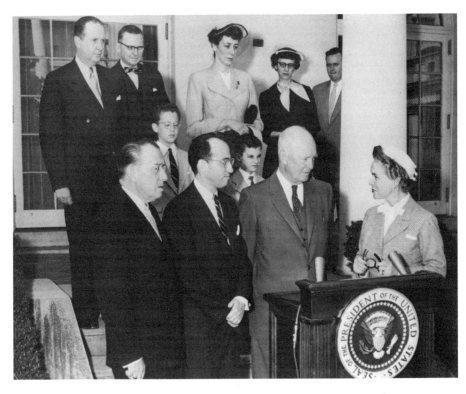

Dr. Salk went to the White House to receive a citation from President Eisenhower.

which forbade patents on results of its research grants. He never made any money from the sale or use of the polio vaccine.

As the vaccine became available, lines of young people formed at the immunization centers. Children were the most common victims of polio and they would get the vaccine first. Until everyone under the age of twenty had been inoculated, no adults except pregnant women (who are especially susceptible to paralytic polio) would be vaccinated.

In reality polio wasn't as deadly as the public believed. Of the 332,835 cases reported in the ten years between 1945 and 1955, 50 percent of the patients recovered completely. Another 30 percent suffered from minor paralysis, while 14 percent of polio victims were severely paralyzed. The disease was fatal in 6 percent of the cases.[3]

Even though polio was not usually fatal, people were terrified of the disease because it left so many young children with permanent injuries. Introduction of the vaccine brought relief to parents because now something could finally be done to stop the terror.

The relief lasted only a short time though. By the end of April grim statistics began to appear. A six-year-old boy in California who had been vaccinated five days earlier suddenly had polio. A toddler in Idaho got polio eight days after his inoculation. Then two little girls died, both after getting shots of the polio vaccine.[4]

Day by day the list of victims grew. Suspension of

the vaccination program was recommended by the government until the source of the infections could be located. Quick detective work traced all of the polio cases to vaccine manufactured by Cutter Laboratories. Cutter's vaccine was recalled, but that didn't end the fear that gripped parents.

The incubation period for polio was from three to thirty-five days, and thousands of children had already received vaccines produced by Cutter Laboratories. For the next several weeks terrified parents watched their sons and daughters for signs of polio. Every headache and fever seemed to be a potential case of the disease.

Finally the incubation period ended and most of those affected could breathe easier. Unfortunately a total of 204 cases of polio occurred that were related to the Cutter product. Dr. Louis Gebhardt of the University of Utah found infectious virus in the samples of Cutter vaccine that he tested.[5]

Jonas Salk said from the beginning that large laboratories might not be as careful as he and his staff had been when they produced the vaccine. During the massive field trial of 1954, every single batch of vaccine was tested by three different laboratories, including Salk's own. After the vaccine was licensed and needed in huge quantities, the testing procedures were much less strict. Only the manufacturer was responsible for safety tests, and the government made random checks on the finished vaccine supply.

Salk wanted the Public Health Service to monitor the manufacturers more closely. He felt that each company needed to prove that it could consistently produce polio vaccine that was free of live viruses. Instead the large companies only reported on the batches of vaccine that they found to be safe. They were not asked to report on how often they found live virus and had to throw the mixture away. Their rate of successful batches of vaccine could not be accurately measured.[6]

Officials realized too late that regulations were inadequate and were not preventing the kind of carelessness that had occurred at Cutter Laboratories. If the immunization program were to continue, all of the procedures and records would have to be examined in the remaining five laboratories.

First Parke, Davis & Company was checked because its polio vaccine department had not experienced any problems in the past. Its records were found to be in order and the company was advised to begin manufacturing the vaccine again. After careful studies were done, vaccine from the other companies was also declared safe. The immunization program would resume. Salk's detailed instructions for producing the vaccine were reviewed, and the five remaining manufacturers were cautioned that they must follow each step exactly as it was outlined.

The public was still somewhat wary, but fear of polio was greater than fear of getting a tainted vaccine.

Demand for the shots soon outgrew the supply since Cutter was no longer making any polio vaccine. Production was increased until eventually everyone who wanted to be vaccinated was finally able to get the shots.

The terrible disease of polio that was once feared by millions slowly lost its power—thanks to the new vaccine. The number of new cases reported in the United States dropped dramatically to 5,485 in 1957 and even farther to 1,300 in 1961—down from 57,879 in 1952.[7]

During 1961 the Surgeon General of the United States licensed a live virus vaccine developed by Dr. Albert Sabin, Salk's former critic. Even though polio seemed to be nearly under control, Sabin believed that Salk's vaccine would not confer lifetime immunity. He convinced the government that only his live virus vaccine would eliminate all polio.

Sabin's vaccine could be given by mouth in drops that were placed on a sugar cube or in a spoon. Once again the public lined up and got a series of three doses of oral polio vaccine that were spaced a month apart. Even those who had already been inoculated with Salk's vaccine wanted to get the new one, too, just to be sure. Questions arose about which vaccine was best. The Public Health Service declared that both were effective. Since Sabin's oral vaccine was easier to take and did not include the use of needles, it became the more popular one in the years ahead.

But Salk said that using a live but weakened virus

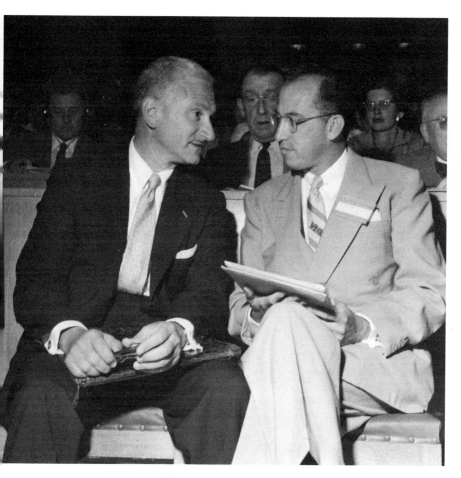

Dr. Salk (right) chats with his most vocal critic, Dr. Albert Sabin. In 1961, Sabin's live polio vaccine was licensed for use.

was dangerous and might cause polio. Why take the chance when the Salk vaccine was effective and safe? More than one hundred cases of paralytic polio were reported after Sabin's vaccine was given. Most of the infections were in adults who had not been previously vaccinated with Salk's product. The adult public was cautioned that the new vaccine might be dangerous for those over eighteen years of age.

Also Sabin's vaccine contains weakened polio virus that multiplies for several weeks in the digestive tract of those who have been immunized. During that time it can sometimes be transmitted by mouth or through feces to unvaccinated people who come into contact with the weakened virus. They can indirectly become immunized in a process known as "herd immunity."[8]

Unfortunately several times a year the live virus in a dose of Sabin's vaccine returns to its original strength or virulence and causes polio. The six to ten cases of the disease that are seen in the United States every year appear to be associated with the Sabin oral vaccine.[9]

After the Cutter incident no cases of polio were linked to Salk's vaccine, which is still used today in many parts of the world. It is easily combined with the routine diphtheria, pertussis, and tetanus (DPT) shots that children get so that a separate injection is not necessary. Tests and follow-up studies also showed that Salk's vaccine did, indeed, produce lifetime immunity after an effective dose was given.[10]

In spite of the fact that Jonas Salk developed the first successful polio vaccine, many of his fellow scientists didn't seem to respect him. During the 1950s a great deal of publicity surrounded the vaccine, and Salk was often at the center of it all. He was a good public speaker and was able to explain how the vaccine worked so that people understood. They liked to listen to him, and he was interviewed often.

Salk's critics accused him of taking advantage of the situation to further his career. In the eyes of some of his peers, Salk merely took Enders's Nobel-Prize-winning work and expanded it. Albert Sabin said that "it was pure kitchen chemistry. Salk didn't discover anything."[11]

At the time that Jonas Salk developed his polio vaccine, much of the basic science and even the technology was there for anyone to use. But Salk was the only researcher of his day who took advantage of Enders's discovery and used the new methods for growing polio virus to create a vaccine that worked.

Many of Salk's critics dismissed the project as scientifically uninteresting. Certainly the research was tedious and repetitious—but necessary for the development of a safe and effective vaccine. Salk alone undertook the massive experiment and effectively brought an end to the polio epidemics that had held the nation in their grip since 1916.

11

After the Vaccine

When all of the confusion finally died down, Dr. Jonas Salk returned to his laboratory in Pittsburgh to resume his work. His interest turned to cancer and its effect on the body's immune system. The University of Pittsburgh was anxious to reward its famous employee for all of the attention he brought to the institution.

It began by changing the name of Municipal Hospital to Salk Hall. Dr. Salk was made Professor of Experimental Medicine, and there were discussions about the formation of a new department for him to run. That department was never established because Jonas Salk's thoughts had begun to turn in a different direction.

Much of his time during the past few years had been consumed by fund-raising, meetings, and speeches. Salk dreamed of a perfect place where scientists could think and do research, away from the pressures of politics and the business world. He didn't imagine a university setting with its obligations to classes and exams either.

The freedom to do nothing but pure research was what Salk had in mind when he talked to his old friend Basil O'Connor, who continued to serve as NFIP president. O'Connor saw the beauty of Salk's plan and agreed to build a research institution with NFIP money if an acceptable site could be found.

After looking at many pieces of property, Salk located a wonderful tract of land that overlooked the Pacific Ocean in La Jolla, California. The shimmering movement of the water would help to provide an atmosphere of serenity and beauty to his community of scholars. The city of San Diego donated the property for the project, and architect Louis Kahn was hired in 1959 to design the buildings.

For the next few years Salk worked closely with Kahn on the center. Eventually two buildings were constructed on the twenty-seven-acre tract of land. The dramatic structures faced each other across a courtyard of concrete. The expanse was divided by a small river of water that stretched toward a perfect backdrop, the Pacific Ocean. The Salk Institute for Biological Studies opened in 1963 with Dr. Salk as its Founding Director. NFIP money financed the construction project as well as

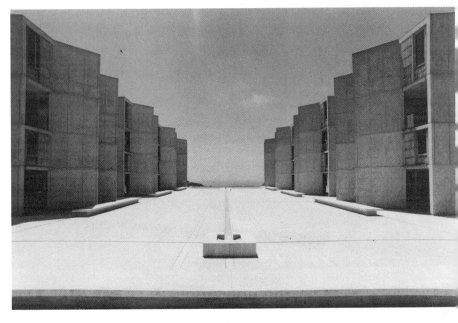

The Salk Institute for Biological Studies is in La Jolla, California.

much of the early operating expenses, and continues to provide $1 million annually to the institute's budget.[1]

Salk and his scientists were involved in some very important work during the next few years. They studied cancer and how the body defends itself against this tragic disease. Multiple sclerosis and autoimmune diseases were also subjects of analysis, as were the brain and peripheral nervous system. Dozens of research papers were written, and the Salk Institute became highly respected in the scientific community.[2]

Within the walls of the institute, however, life was less than perfect. Funding and administrative problems surfaced and had to be solved. Jonas Salk's personal life was also falling apart, and he and Donna divorced in 1968. As the years passed and he grew older, Jonas Salk began to view his work a little differently.

No longer was the world of pure science foremost in his mind. He was now concerned not only with the health of the world's people, but also with people's ability to adapt to a changing environment of pollution and overpopulation. He wrote of his concerns about the quality of life in several philosophical books titled *The Anatomy of Reality, World Population and Human Values, The Survival of the Wisest,* and *Man Unfolding.*[3]

In 1970 Dr. Jonas Salk married a painter named Francoise Gilot. She had spent many years with the famous artist Pablo Picasso and is the author of the book *My Life With Picasso.* Today the couple lives in a house built on a cliff that rises 600 feet above the Pacific Ocean.

During his long career Salk has held many advisory positions such as Consultant to the Secretary of the Army in Epidemic Diseases during the years 1947–1954. He has also been given numerous awards, including a Congressional Gold Medal in 1955 and the Presidential Medal of Freedom in 1977. In 1986 he became a member of the California AIDS Vaccine Research and Development Advisory Committee. AIDS stands for acquired immunodeficiency syndrome.

In recent years Salk has focused his attention on a vaccine to prevent AIDS, a killer of immense proportions. As in the days of polio, the world is desperate for something that will stop the dreaded disease.

In 1987 Jonas Salk and his associates began work on an AIDS vaccine. Their laboratories are not at the Salk Institute, but instead, at the Immune Response Corporation located in nearby San Diego. They are applying Salk's old successful methods and using an inactivated virus in an attempt to create a vaccine to fight AIDS.

Salk's plans include a dual approach to the problem. First he wants to develop a vaccine for people who have already tested positive for the human immunodeficiency virus (HIV), which leads to AIDS. He hopes that his vaccine will improve the victim's immune system so that

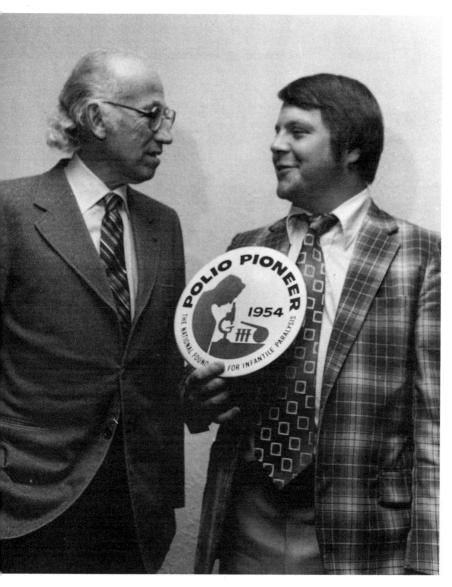

Dr. Salk and "Polio Pioneer," Randy Kerr, met for the first time in 1980.

AIDS never develops. If his immunotherapy succeeds, then infected people might be able to lead relatively normal lives even though they are HIV-positive.

Salk's second approach involves a vaccine that would actually prevent infection by HIV just as the polio vaccine prevents infection by polio viruses. When the time arrives to test this vaccine, Jonas Salk plans to use himself as a guinea pig, just as he did with his experimental polio vaccine.[4]

Many researchers around the world are also engaged in experiments in the race to find a cure for AIDS. Some are working with the entire inactivated virus as Salk is. But more often only parts of the virus are being used in the production of candidate vaccines. Many scientists feel that it is too risky to inject the entire virus into people, in spite of the fact that it has been inactivated.

Even if Salk succeeds and creates an AIDS vaccine, it may only be effective in some parts of the world. Since the virus constantly changes, or mutates, the disease that is seen in the United States may not be exactly the same as the one that infects people in Africa or China.

At the Immune Response Corporation the mysteries surrounding AIDS have been under intense investigation for several years. Monkeys have once again proven to be valuable tools in the search for a vaccine. Because monkeys are susceptible to a disease similar to AIDS, caused by simian immunodeficiency virus (SIV), they make good laboratory subjects.

Monkeys also develop the disease at a much faster rate than humans. Data from the animal experiments can be compiled in a few months instead of several years. Chimpanzees are the best test animals, since they can actually be infected with HIV rather than SIV.[5] However, chimpanzees are an endangered species, and they are only available in small numbers for laboratory experiments.

Jonas Salk and his associates tested a vaccine on chimps infected with HIV and found no sign of the virus in later blood samples. They then moved on to a small group of HIV-positive human volunteers and administered the vaccine to them. In the human subjects, the vaccine did not cause the disease to progress any faster, and it produced an immune response in some of the patients. However many more tests and volunteers must be studied before any definite conclusions can be drawn.[6]

As Salk and other AIDS researchers continue their battle against this killer, millions of HIV-infected people all over the world wait. The virus is spreading at an alarming rate and shows no signs of slowing down. The world's hope lies with scientists like Jonas Salk, who have a mission and will not stop their work until a vaccine is found.

Polio and Salk
in the 1990s

In its day polio was as frightening to the world's people as AIDS is today. Efforts to eliminate polio in the United States were very successful. Except for a handful of cases a year that are usually associated with the Sabin vaccine, polio is a disease of the past. In the Western Hemisphere a few cases still occur, but the number has dropped rapidly.

Massive vaccination programs in Central and South America during the past few years have been very effective. In other areas of the world such as India, Africa, and China, polio is still a serious threat. There are as many as 185,000 cases reported every year. WHO wants to try to eliminate polio from the entire planet by the year 2000.[1]

Even though new cases of the disease very rarely

occur today in the United States, polio is still the cause of much suffering. There are an estimated 650,000 survivors of the epidemics of the 1940s and 1950s. Many of them have spent their lives disabled to varying degrees and must use crutches, braces, and sometimes wheelchairs to get around.[2]

Other polio survivors have less severe disabilities, and until recently, some suffered very little after they recovered from their initial illness. Unfortunately new worries have begun to surface during the past few years. Some former polio patients have started to experience extreme fatigue, followed several months later by muscle weakness, joint pain, and breathing and swallowing problems.

A former patient may stumble or trip more often or have problems going up and down stairs. Difficulties may be encountered during long periods of writing or drawing if the arms were affected by the initial infection. In the beginning doctors thought that their patients were experiencing the normal problems that are associated with getting older. But as more and more people reported similar symptoms, the medical community began to see a pattern. Studies showed that the complaints were often related to an earlier polio infection. As many as half of all former patients were found to be experiencing aftereffects of the original infection as many as twenty-five and forty years later.[3]

Researchers found that motor nerve cells that were

initially spared by polio were apparently wearing out at a faster rate than normal as the patient aged. These nerves had taken over for the ones destroyed by the virus. Messages sent from the brain had a harder time reaching the muscles via the overused nerve cells. The result was a feeling of weakness in the legs, arms, and muscles involved in breathing and swallowing.[4]

The name Post Polio Syndrome (PPS) was given to the array of symptoms experienced by former polio patients. Therapy includes frequent rest periods, weight control, and moderate exercise such as swimming. Those who must once again use braces to support weakened limbs, however, find that today each device weighs only two to three pounds instead of the fifteen-pound braces of the past.[5]

Unfortunately all former polio patients are at some risk for developing the syndrome. It seems that those who suffered with the disease in the past may not be finished with it even today. Without the efforts of Jonas Salk forty years ago there would certainly be many thousands more people at risk for developing PPS.

Even though he is approaching eighty years of age, Dr. Salk has never considered retirement. He continues to work a staggering number of hours each day in his search for an AIDS vaccine. Sometimes after a long day's work, Salk gets up in the middle of the night to record the thoughts circulating in his mind. The ideas that he has are a mixture of dreams and reality, and he writes them down in simple spiral notebooks like the ones students carry.

In the pages of his notebooks are records of his connection to what he sometimes calls the "cosmic consciousness." He believes that there is a greater knowledge or energy force that is sometimes available to those who are fortunate enough to discover it. He feels that all of his past work has been a result of the influence of this power and that his future work will be guided by it as well.[6]

The Salk Institute currently employs 500 scientists and staff members and is responsible for an impressive body of work. Salk himself is the Founding Director of the institute and the author of more than 135 scientific papers. He is a member of numerous organizations that include the Academy of Arts and Sciences, the American Public Health Association, and Physicians for Social Responsibility.

His lifelong interest in immunization led him to join a group of fellow scientists in 1986 to study childhood illnesses. Polio and other preventable infectious diseases still pose a serious threat in some parts of the world. Doctor Salk and his associates are working to encourage vaccination programs that will help to eliminate many preventable conditions in underdeveloped countries.[7]

In addition to his own busy schedule, Jonas Salk proudly follows the medical careers of his three sons. Peter, the oldest, is involved in AIDS research with his father. Darrell spent some years as a pediatrician, but now does research in the area of cancer diagnosis and treatment. Salk's youngest son Jonathan is a psychiatrist. In keeping with the family trend of producing only male heirs, the Salk brothers have provided their father with four grandsons.[8]

Hopefully his grandsons' generation will also be blessed with dedicated men and women who strive to make all of our lives better. Jonas Salk has certainly made major contributions in his lifetime and he is not yet finished.

Maybe the children of tomorrow will view the AIDS pandemic with detachment and curiosity the way the children of today view polio. Perhaps AIDS will simply be a historical event that has been almost forgotten by everyone except those who suffered through it. When a disease such as polio or AIDS becomes just a bad memory, that is the greatest tribute that can be paid to a scientist such as Dr. Jonas Salk.

Chronology

1914—Jonas Salk born on October 28 in New York City.

1916—First polio epidemic in the United States.

1918—Twenty-two million die worldwide in influenza pandemic.

1921—Future President Franklin Roosevelt infected with polio.

1929—Salk graduates Townsend Harris High School at age fifteen, then enters City College of New York.

1934—Salk graduates City College, then begins medical school at New York University School of Medicine.

1938—President Roosevelt establishes National Foundation for Infantile Paralysis (NFIP).

1939—Salk graduates medical school on June 8; marries Donna Lindsay on June 9.

1942—Salk begins work for Dr. Thomas Francis at the University of Michigan.

1944—Son Peter born.

1947—Son Darrell born; Salk begins work at the University of Pittsburgh.

1949—Enders grows polio virus in non-nervous tissue; Salk begins polio virus typing program.

1950—Son Jonathan born.

1952—Salk tests polio vaccine at the Watson Home.

1954—Nationwide field trial of Salk vaccine conducted.

1955—Salk vaccine licensed by the U.S. government.

1956—Salk receives first Congressional Medal for Distinguished Civilian Service.

1961—Sabin oral vaccine licensed by the U.S. government.

1963—Salk Institute opens in La Jolla, California.

1968—Salk and wife Donna divorce.

1970—Salk marries artist Francoise Gilot.

1977—Salk receives Presidential Medal of Freedom.

1987—Salk begins work on AIDS vaccine.

1992—Salk's experimental AIDS vaccine produces an immune response in some HIV-infected human volunteers.

Chapter Notes

Chapter 1

1. "It Works," *Time,* April 25, 1955, pp. 50–52.

Chapter 2

1. Dorothy and Philip Sterling, *Polio Pioneers* (Garden City, NY: Doubleday & Company, Inc., 1955), p. 15.

2. Richard Carter, *Breakthrough: The Saga of Jonas Salk* (New York: Trident Press, 1966), p. 3.

Chapter 3

1. Jack Fincher, "America's Deadly Rendezvous with the Spanish Lady," *Smithsonian,* January 1989, p. 140.

2. Fincher, p. 132.

3. Tom Gyurik, Public Health Advisor, Centers for Disease Control—Influenza Division.

4. Joan Goldberg, "The Creative Mind," *Science Digest,* June 1984, pp. 51–52.

5. Jane Smith, *Patenting the Sun* (New York: William Morrow and Company, 1990), p. 96.

Chapter 4

1. "Smallpox," *Academic American Encyclopedia* (Grolier Electronic Publishing, Inc., 1991).

Chapter 5

1. Richard Carter, *Breakthrough: The Saga of Jonas Salk* (New York: Trident Press, 1966), p. 14.

Chapter 6

1. "Poliomyelitis," *Encyclopaedia Britannica* (Chicago: Encyclopaedia Britannica, Inc., 1974), vol. 8, p. 81.

2. Interview with George Trader, hospital administrator, March 1992.

3. Interview with Eddie Rosenwasser, paralyzed bulbar polio victim, April 22, 1992.

4. Interview with George Trader, hospital administrator, March 1992.

5. *Encyclopaedia Britannica,* p. 81.

Chapter 7

1. Aaron Klein, *Trial by Fury* (New York: Charles Scribner's Sons, 1972), p. 52.

2. "Closing in on Polio," *Time,* March 29, 1954, pp. 56–65.

3. Richard Carter, *Breakthrough: The Saga of Jonas Salk* (New York: Trident Press, 1966), p. 79.

4. *Time,* March 29, 1954, p. 56.

5. "Vaccine Evidence," *Time,* May 23, 1955, pp. 48–49.

Chapter 8

1. Jane Smith, *Patenting the Sun* (New York: William Morrow and Company, 1990), p. 136.

2. "U.S. Polio Survivors: The Numbers From Two Sources," *Polio Network News,* Winter 1991, p. 4.

Chapter 9

1. Richard Carter, *Breakthrough: The Saga of Jonas Salk* (New York: Trident Press, 1966), p. 97.

2. "Polio Pioneers," *Time,* April 26, 1954, p. 53.

3. Jane Smith, *Patenting the Sun* (New York: William Morrow and Company, 1990), p. 273.

4. Aaron Klein, *Trial By Fury* (New York: Charles Scribner's Sons, 1972), p. 102.

5. "It Works," *Time,* April 25, 1955, pp. 50–52.

Chapter 10

1. "A Quiet Young Man's Magnificent Victory," *Newsweek,* April 25, 1955, pp. 64–67.

2. "It Works," *Time,* April 25, 1955, p. 51.

3. "The Polio Scramble," *Newsweek,* May 2, 1955, pp. 79–81.

4. "Vaccine Crisis," *Time,* May 9, 1955, p. 56.

5. "Questions Without Answers," *Time,* June 20, 1955, p. 67.

6. "Premature and Crippled," *Time,* June 20, 1955, pp. 45–46.

7. "Why There's Worry Over Polio Vaccine," *U.S. News and World Report,* October 19, 1964, p. 12.

8. Rick Weiss, "Polio Policy: A Bitter Pill to Swallow," *Science News,* July 16, 1988, p. 43.

9. Joan Goldberg, "The Creative Mind," *Science Digest,* June 1984, p. 51.

10. Telephone interview with Jonas Salk, June 23, 1992.

11. George Johnson, "Once Again a Man with a Mission," *The New York Times Magazine,* November 25, 1990, pp. 57–61.

Chapter 11

1. Ellen Posner, "Louis Kahn's High Aesthetic Calling," *The Atlantic,* October 1991, pp. 114–122.

2. Peter Stoler, "A Conversation with Jonas Salk," *Psychology Today,* March 1983, pp. 50–56.

3. James Reston, Jr., "Interview: Jonas Salk," *Omni,* May 1982, pp. 97–104.

4. Telephone interview with Jonas Salk, April 22, 1992.

5. Peter Radetsky, "Closing in on an AIDS Vaccine," *Discover,* September 1990, pp. 71–77.

6. Telephone interview with Jonas Salk, April 22, 1992.

Chapter 12

1. Teri Randall, "Rest of World Ready to Follow This Hemisphere's Approach to Eliminating Polio in Near Future," *The Journal of the American Medical Association,* February 20, 1991, pp. 839–840.

2. "The Late Effects of Polio: An Overview," International Polio Network Pamphlet, St. Louis, Missouri.

3. Marny Eulberg, M.D.; Lauro Halstead, M.D.; and Jacquelin Perry, M.D., "Post Polio Syndrome: How You Can Help," *Patient Care,* June 15, 1988, p. 131.

4. Theodore Munsat, M.D., "Poliomyelitis—New Problems with an Old Disease," *The New England Journal of Medicine,* April 25, 1991, pp. 1206–1207.

5. Eulberg et al., p. 131.

6. George Johnson, "Once Again a Man with a Mission," *The New York Times,* p. 60.

7. "Jonas Salk Biographical Sketch," The Salk Institute, 5 pp.

8. Telephone interview with Jonas Salk, April 22, 1992.

Further Reading

Crofford, Emily. *Healing Warrior: A Story About Sister Elizabeth Kenny.* Minneapolis: Carolrhoda, 1989.

Fincher, Jack. "America's Deadly Rendezvous with the Spanish Lady." *Smithsonian,* January 1989, pp. 131–145.

Gallagher, Hugh. *FDR's Splendid Deception.* New York: Dodd, Mead, 1985.

Gallo, Robert, MD. *Virus Hunting.* New York: Harper Collins, 1991.

Hall, Robert. *Through the Storm: A Polio Story.* St. Cloud, Minn.: North Star Press of St. Cloud, Inc., 1990.

Johnson, George. "Once Again a Man with a Mission." *The New York Times Magazine,* November 25, 1990, pp. 57–61.

Klein, Aaron. *Trial by Fury.* New York: Charles Scribner's Sons, 1972.

Radetsky, Peter. "Closing in on an AIDS Vaccine." *Discover,* September, 1990, pp. 71–77.

Silverstein, Alvin, Virginia Silverstein, and Robert Silverstein. *AIDS: Deadly Threat.* Hillside, N.J. Enslow, 1991.

Smith, Jane. *Patenting the Sun.* New York: William Morrow and Company, 1990.

Weiss, Rick. "Polio Policy: A Bitter Pill to Swallow." *Science News,* July 16, 1988, p. 43.

Index

About the Author

Carmen Bredeson, a former high school English teacher, received her master's degree in instructional technology. In addition to fundraising and performing volunteer work for public libraries, Ms. Bredeson now devotes much of her time to writing. A mother of two, she lives with her family in Texas.